# WALL PILATE

# WORKOUTS

## FOR WOMEN

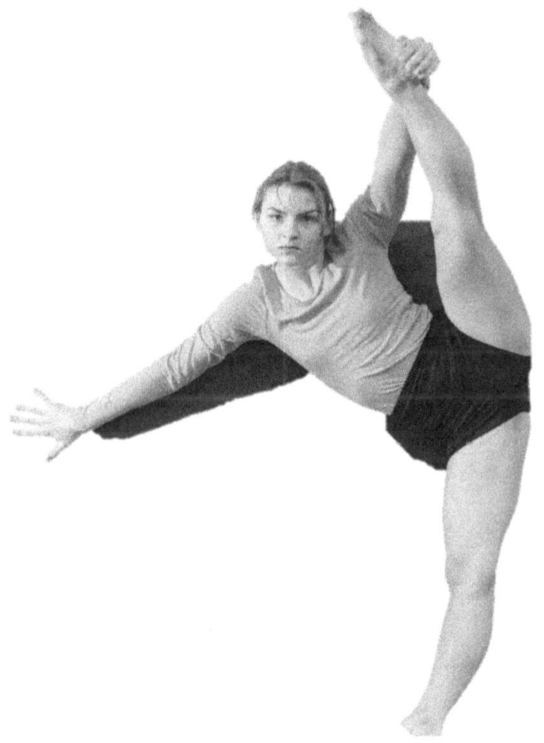

## Jesus Mendez

# TABLE OF CONTENT

"The only bad
workout is the one
that didn't happen."
– Unknown

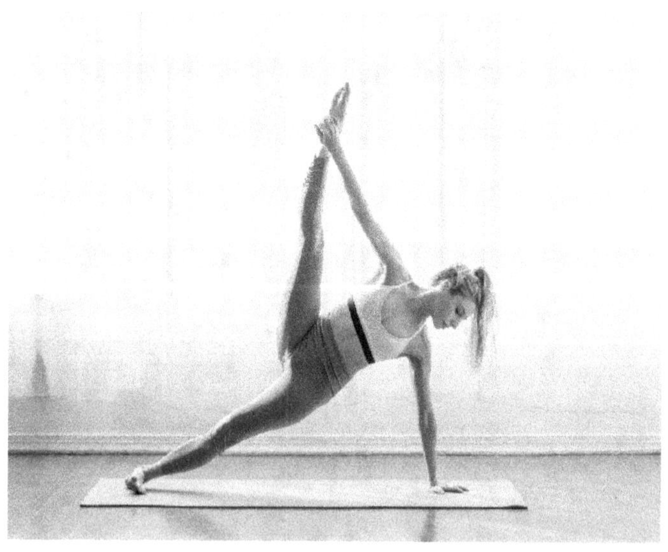

# INTRODUCTION

Meet Joyce, a vibrant lady who, like many others, desired a workout program that worked with her hectic lifestyle. Joyce was blown away by the transforming impact of consistency two weeks into her encounter with wall Pilates.

Joyce carved out times with the wall as her constant friend in the early mornings, amidst the symphony of singing birds. Initially hesitant, she accepted the advice, finding consolation in the seamless combination of challenge and support provided by this one-of-a-kind activity. The tiny alterations grew into noticeable leaps of change as the days progressed.

Her muscles, which had formerly muttered objections, now echoed resilience, shaped by the many motions against the dependable wall. She built a stronger core and discovered unknown flexibility with each elegant stretch and intentional engagement. The wall became more than just a barrier; it became an ally, a quiet confidante on her thrilling adventure.

Joyce's story demonstrates the tremendous transformation that occurs when determination meets a specific program. Her journey emphasizes the possibility that exists inside the boundaries of constancy, commitment, and the embracing of a revolutionary workout program.

# Chapter One

## Setting the Foundation

**"Strength doesn't come from what you can do; it comes from overcoming the things you once thought you couldn't." - Rikki Rogers**

## Introduction to Wall Pilates for Women

Wall Pilates is a versatile and efficient technique for women to supplement their home workout regimens. It is designed to increase core strength, flexibility, and muscular tone overall. The wall acts as a supporting tool for various activities, making them accessible to people of all fitness levels.

## 2. The Importance of Correct Form and Alignment

In each exercise, emphasize the importance of maintaining appropriate form and alignment. Correct posture not only increases the advantages of the workout, but it also decreases the danger of strain or injury. Encourage practitioners to use their core muscles and maintain a neutral body alignment.

• Keep the head, shoulders, and hips in a straight line to align the spine.

• Draw the navel towards the spine to engage the core muscles.

• Avoid overhanging or rounding the back; keep it natural.

## 3. Space Preparation: Clearing and Preparing the Wall Area

Make a free area against a wall before beginning the workout. Check for any adjacent obstructions or sharp items. During floor-based activities, a yoga mat or padded surface might give comfort.

• Select a clean and clutter-free wall area, ideally without any wall hangings or impediments.

• To cushion the spine during floor activities, use a yoga mat or a folded towel.

• Keep a water bottle and a towel accessible for hydration and perspiration removal.

## 1. Stretching and Breathing Exercises to Warm Up

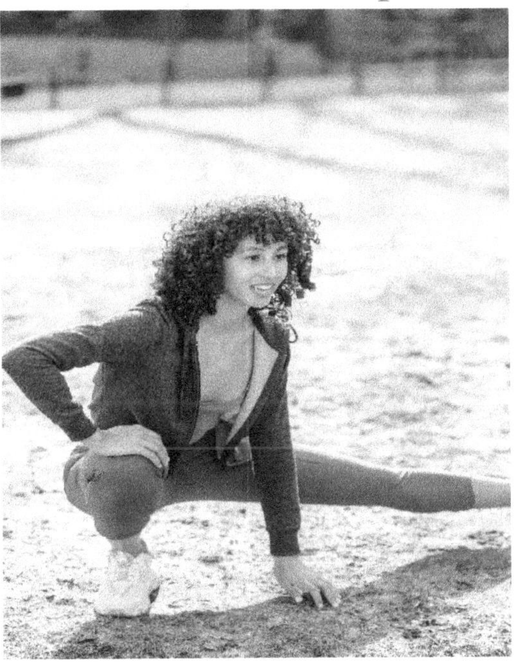

To promote blood flow and flexibility, begin the practice with a series of vigorous warm-up stretches. Include exercises that target main muscle groups and joints, prepping the body for the following workouts. To increase relaxation and attention, combine these stretches with regulated breathing.

## Warm-up

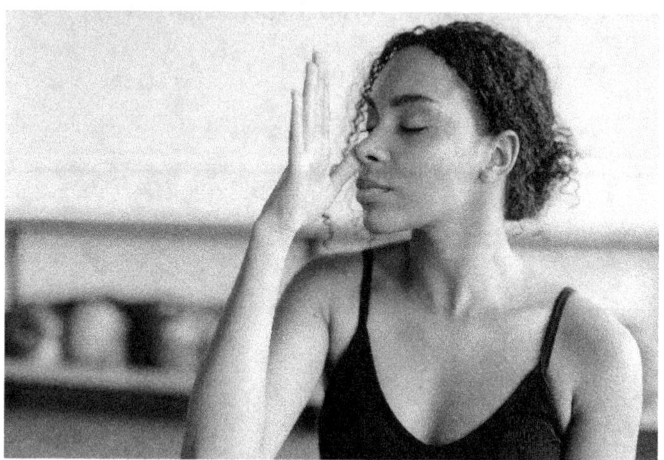

• Neck rotations, shoulder rolls, and arm swings to loosen upper body muscles.

• Leg swings, hip circles, and ankle rotations to loosen lower body muscles.

• Deep breathing techniques: inhale deeply through the nose, exhale fully through the mouth, focusing on relaxation.

"Strength doesn't come from what you can do; it comes from overcoming the things you once thought you couldn't." - Rikki Rogers

# Chapter Two

## Wall Core Strengthening

**"The body achieves what the mind believes." - Not known**

## 1. Investigating Wall Sit-Ups and Leg Raises

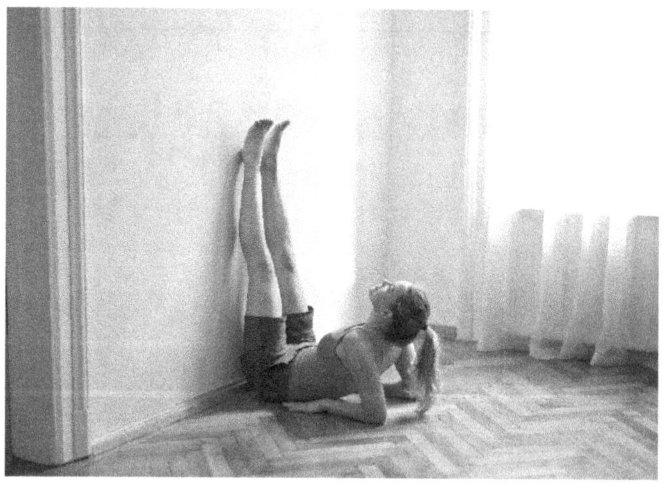

### Wall Sit-Ups

Begin by reclining on the mat with your legs stretched against the wall. Lift your torso slowly towards your knees while engaging your core. Lower yourself back down with control. Aim for 10-15 repetitions.

Lie on your back with your legs against the wall. Lift your legs up and straighten them. Lower them without letting them hit the floor. Perform 10-12 repetitions.

## 2. Wall Supported Plank Variations

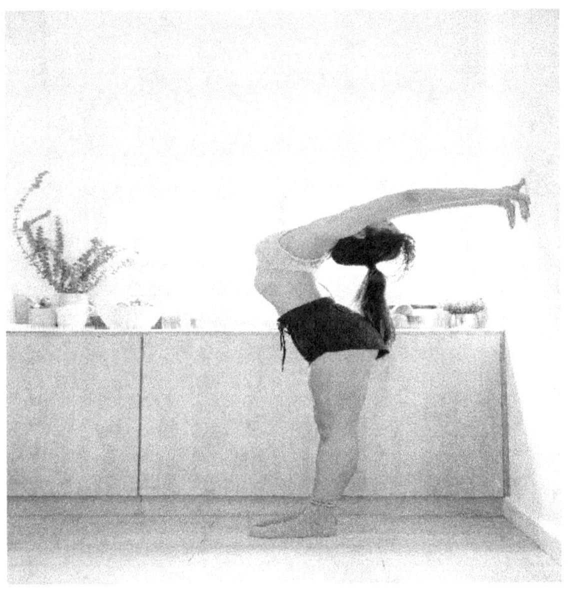

### Wall Plank

Get into a plank posture with your forearms on the floor and your fcct against the wall.

Hold for 30 to 60 seconds, focusing on activating the core muscles.



Create a side plank posture by resting one forearm against the wall. Maintain a straight line from head to feet by lifting your hips off the ground. Hold each side for 20-30 seconds.

## 1. Waist and oblique Strengthening Side Planks

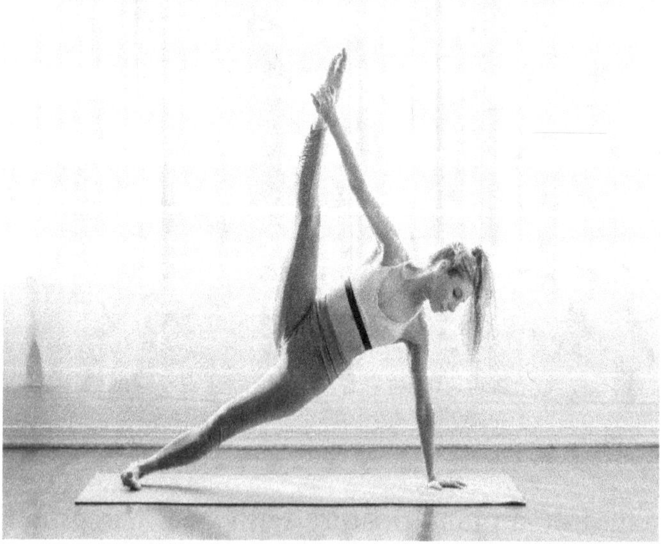

## Wall Side Crunches

Stand with one shoulder against the wall, sideways. Raise your arm overhead. Crunch sideways slowly, bringing the elbow to the hip. Complete 12-15 repetitions on each side.

**4.** Pelvic tilts and abdominal engagement exercises are introduced.

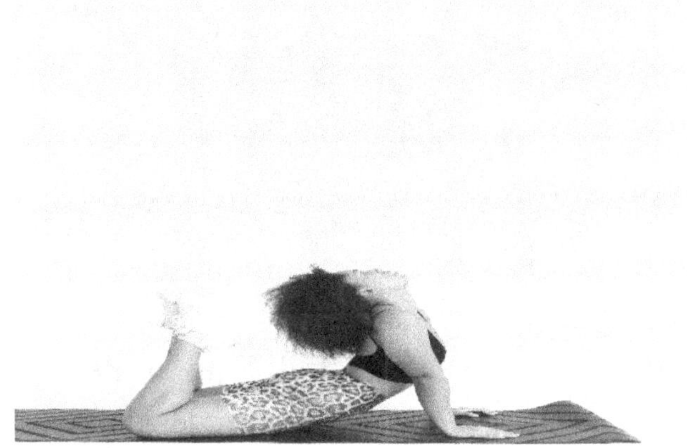

## Pelvic Tilts

Lie down on your back with your knees bent and your feet against a wall. Tilt your pelvis forward and press your lower back against the mat. Hold for a few seconds before releasing. Repeat 10-12 times more.

## Abdominal Engagement

Position yourself with your back to the wall. Pull your belly button towards your spine to engage your core. Hold for 20-30 seconds while breathing normally.

## Conclusion

These exercises focus the core muscles, assisting in strengthening and toning while using a wall for support. Individual fitness levels may be used to vary the repetitions and length of each exercise.

"The body achieves what the mind believes." - Not known

# Chapter Three

## Balance and Flexibility

**"Balance is not something you find, it's something you create." Jana Kingsford's**

## 1. Wall Stretches for Leg Flexibility

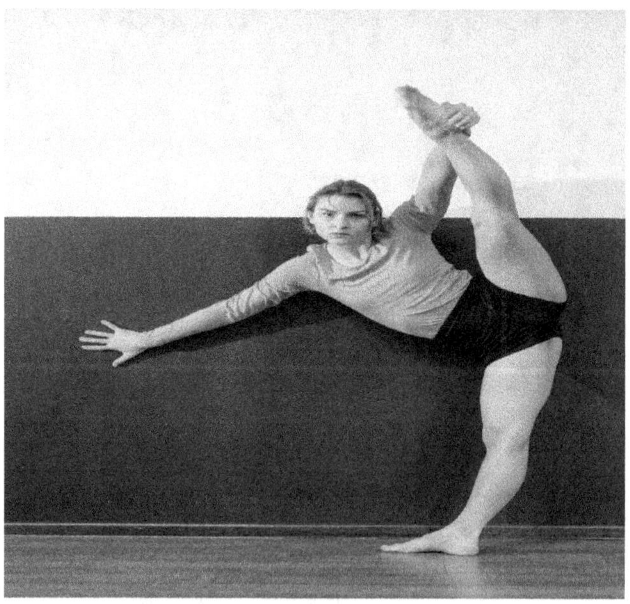

Lie on your back with one leg stretched up
the wall and the other relaxed on the floor
for a hamstring stretch. Pull the outstretched

leg towards you gently, feeling a stretch
down the back of the leg. Hold for 30
seconds before switching sides.

## Quad Stretch

Face the wall and grab on for support. Bend
one leg and bring your foot up to your
glutes. Hold the foot with your hand until
you feel a stretch at the front of your thigh.
Hold each leg for 20-30 seconds.

## 2. Wall Supported Standing Balance Exercises

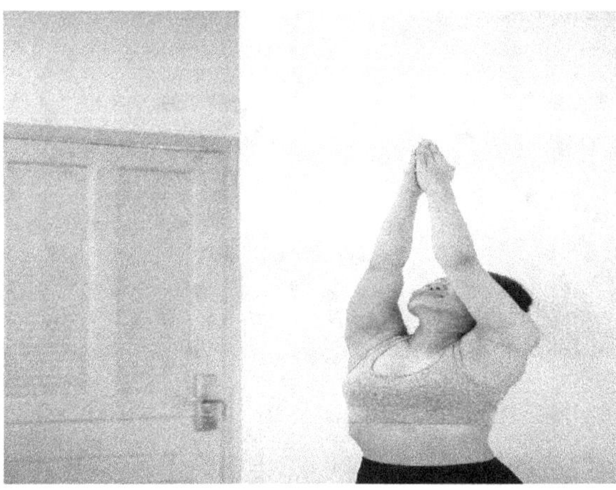

## Single-Leg Balance

Stand near a wall and place a hand on it for support. Lift one foot off the ground while remaining balanced on the other. Hold for 20-30 seconds before alternating legs. Increase the length gradually as your balance improves.

## Tree Pose Variation

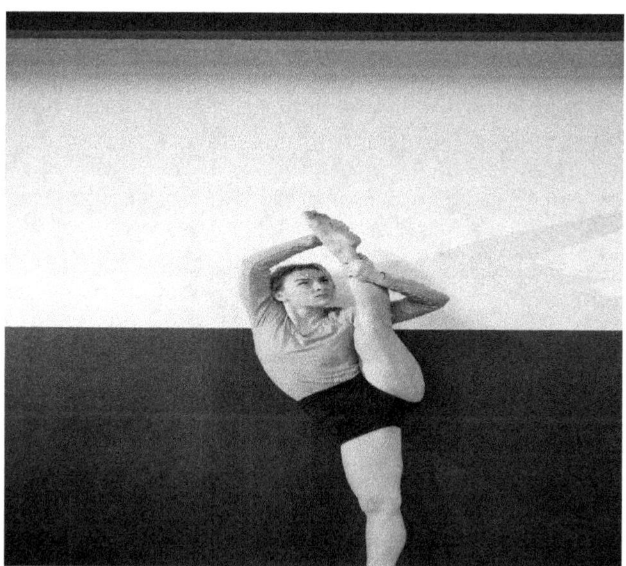

Begin by standing near a wall. Place the sole of one foot on the opposing leg's inner thigh or calf. Find your center of gravity and hold for 20-30 seconds per side.

# Increase Flexibility Through Wall Stretches

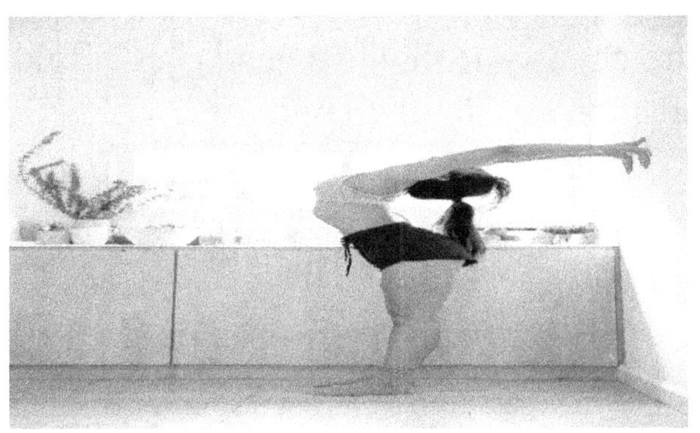

## Wall Pigeon Pose

Lie back against a wall and cross one ankle over the opposing knee. Slide your foot up the wall, feeling the hip and glutes stretch. Hold for 30 seconds before switching sides.

## Wall Cobra Stretch

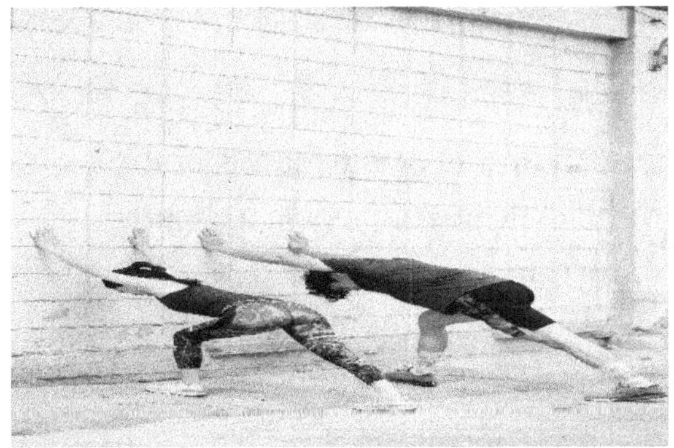

Face the wall and lay your hands at shoulder height on it. Step back and forth, bringing your chest closer to the wall. Feel the stretch in your shoulders and chest. Hold the position for 20-30 seconds.

## Including Yoga-Inspired Wall Poses

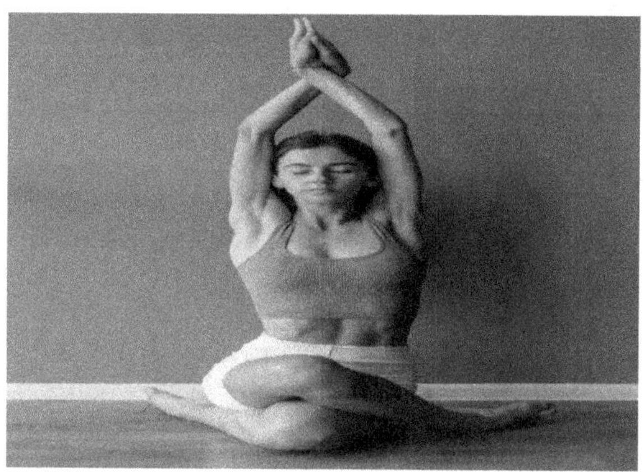

## Wall Supported Downward Dog

Face the wall and lay your hands at hip height on it. Allow your body to bend forward, forming an inverted V shape as you walk backward. Feel the hamstrings and shoulders stretch. Hold the position for 30 seconds.

## Conclusion

These exercises use the wall to help with flexibility and balance while combining components of yoga-inspired positions.

"Balance is not something you find, it's something you create." Jana Kingsford's

# Chapter Four

## Lower Body Focus

**"Your legs are not giving out. Your head is giving up. Keep going." – Unknown**

## Wall Squats and Variations for Lower Body Toning

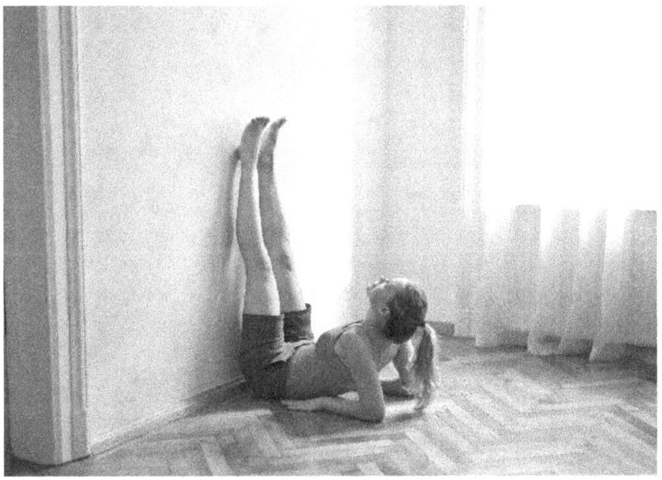

### Wall Squats

Stand with your back against the wall and lower your body into a seated position, as if sitting in an invisible chair. Hold for 20-30 seconds or longer, focusing on engaging the thighs and glutes. Gradually increase hold time as strength improves.

## Pulse Squats

Perform wall squats with a slight variation by pulsing up and down in the seated position. Aim for 10-15 pulses per set.

## Targeting Glutes and Hamstrings with Wall Lunges

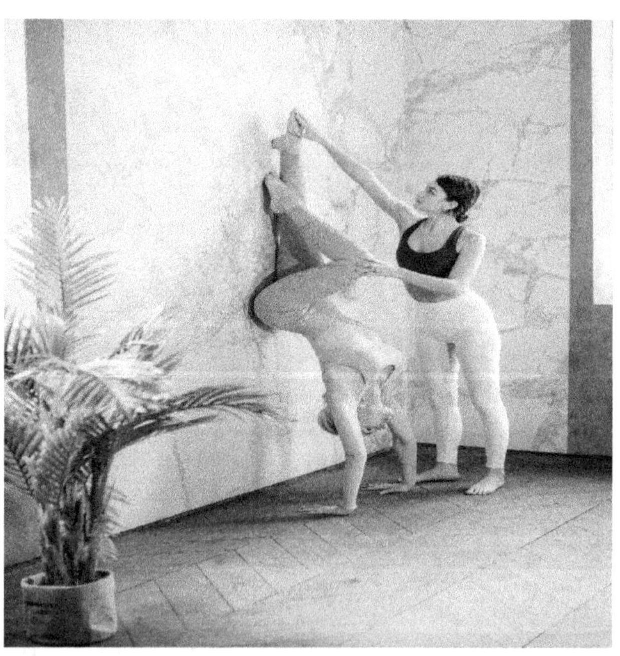

## Reverse Wall Lunges

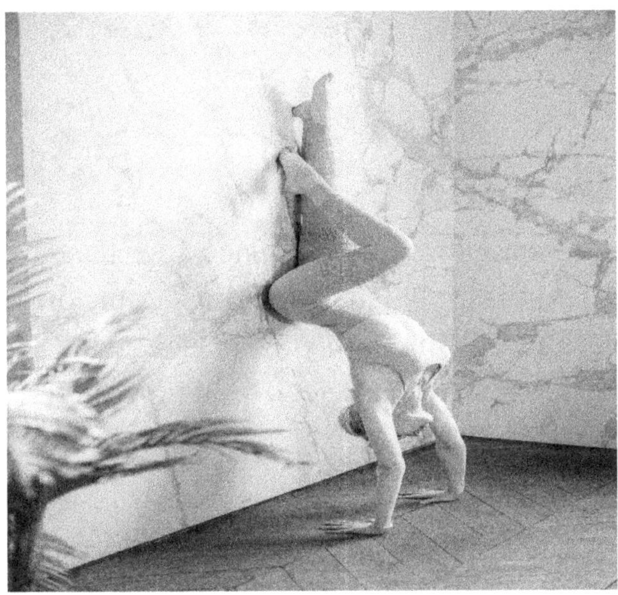

Stand facing away from the wall, hands resting against it for balance. Step back with one leg into a lunge position, bending both knees. Return to the starting position and switch legs. Perform 10-12 reps per leg.

## Wall-Supported Forward Lunges

Stand facing the wall with hands placed on it for support. Step forward into a lunge position, keeping the front knee aligned with the ankle. Return to the starting position and alternate legs. Aim for 10-12 reps per leg.

# Calf Raises and Leg Extensions Using the Wall

## Wall Calf Raises

Stand facing the wall and place your hands lightly on it for balance. Lift your heels off the ground, rising onto your toes. Lower back down and repeat for 15-20 repetitions.

## Wall Leg Extensions

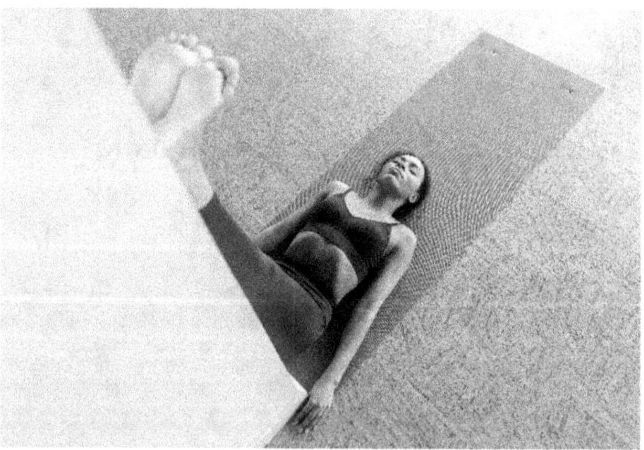

Lie on your back with legs extended upward against the wall. Lower one leg down towards the floor, keeping it straight, then lift it back up. Alternate legs and perform 12-15 reps per leg.

# Cooling Down with Lower Body Stretches

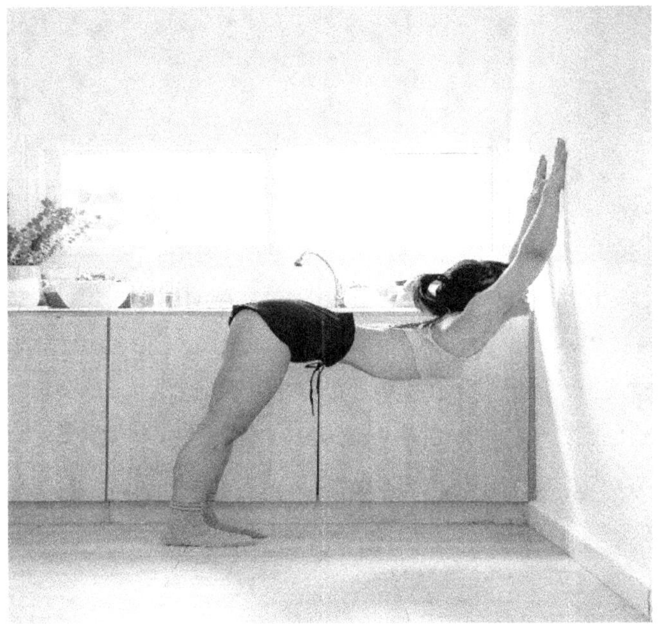

## Wall Supported Quad Stretch

Stand facing the wall and grab one foot, bringing it towards your glutes. Maintain balance by keeping the supporting leg slightly bent. Hold for 20-30 seconds per leg.

*Wall Butterfly Stretch*: Sit facing the wall with the soles of your feet together. Gently press your knees toward the wall, feeling a stretch in your inner thighs. Hold for 30 seconds while breathing deeply.

## Conclusion

These exercises target various muscle groups in the lower body, providing an effective workout while utilizing the support of a wall. Moving forward, I'll detail Chapter 5, which focuses on upper body strengthening exercises.

"Your legs are not giving out. Your head is giving up. Keep going." – Unknown

# Chapter Five

## Upper Body Strengthening

**"The only bad workout is the one that didn't happen." - Unknown**

## Wall Push-Ups and Modifications for Upper Body Strength

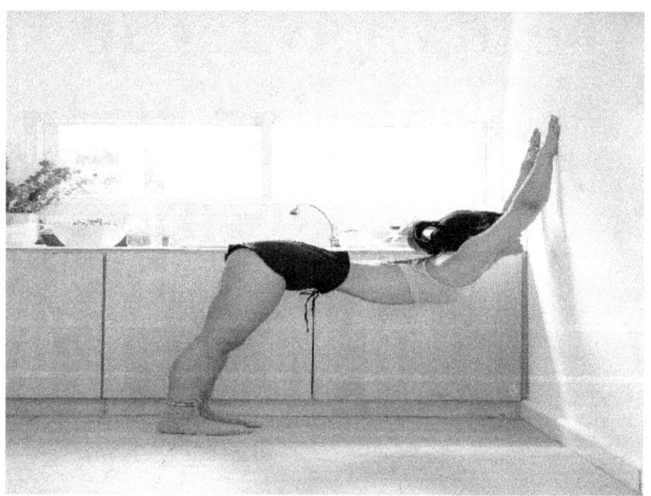

### Wall Push-Ups

Stand facing the wall, arms extended, and hands placed shoulder-width apart. Lower your chest toward the wall by bending your elbows, then push back up. Aim for 12-15 repetitions.

## Incline Push-Ups

Place your hands on the wall wider than shoulder-width apart and perform push-ups. This variation targets different areas of the chest and arms. Aim for 10-12 reps.

## Triceps Dips and Arm Exercises

## Utilizing the Wall

## Wall Triceps Dips

Sit on the floor with your back against the wall, palms on the floor behind you, fingers facing towards your body. Lift your hips off the ground, bending your elbows to lower your body, then straighten your arms to return to the starting position. Aim for 10-12 reps.

*Wall Arm Circles*: Stand facing the wall with arms extended sideways. Make small circles in a forward direction for 20-30 seconds, then reverse the circles for another 20-30 seconds.

# Shoulder Stabilization Exercises

## Against the Wall

### Wall Shoulder Taps

Assume a plank position facing the wall. Lift one hand and touch the opposite shoulder, alternating sides. Aim for 10-12 taps on each shoulder.

### Wall Y Raises

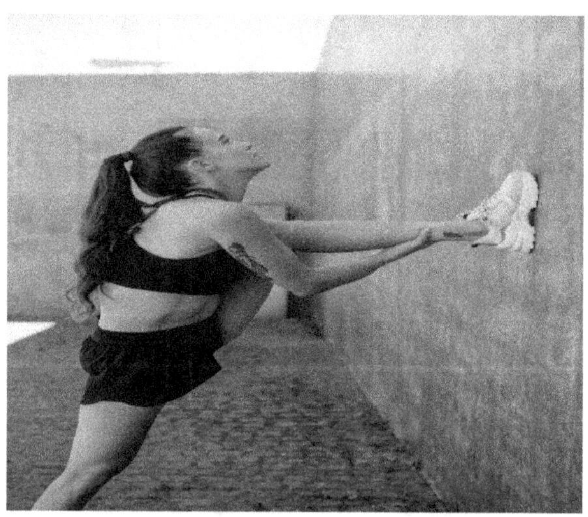

 Stand with your back against the wall, arms extended straight out in a Y shape. Slowly raise your arms up, keeping them straight, and then lower them back down. Aim for 12-15 reps.

## Incorporating Resistance Bands for Added Intensity

## Wall Band Pull-Aparts

Secure a resistance band around a wall fixture or doorknob at chest height. Hold the band with both hands and pull it apart, bringing your hands towards your chest. Return to the starting position and repeat for 12-15 reps.

## Conclusion

These upper body exercises utilize the wall for support and target various muscle groups, enhancing strength and toning. Next, we'll move on to Chapter 6, focusing on combining the exercises into a personalized wall Pilates routine and additional tips for progression and recovery.

"The only bad
workout is the one
that didn't happen."
- Unknown

# Chapter Six

## Putting It All Together

**"Success is the sum of small efforts, repeated day in and day out." - Robert Collier**

## Creating Your Custom Wall Pilates Routine

Combine exercises from previous chapters into a structured workout routine. Design a sequence that targets different muscle groups while considering individual fitness levels and goals. Start with a warm-up, progress through targeted exercises, and conclude with a cool-down.

## Sample Routine:

- Warm-up stretches: 5 minutes
- Core exercises: 10-15 minutes
- Flexibility and balance: 10 minutes
- Lower body focus: 10-15 minutes

- Upper body strengthening: 10-15 minutes
- Cool-down stretches: 5-10 minutes

## Tips for Progression and Increasing Difficulty

Gradually increase the intensity by incorporating variations, increasing repetitions or hold times, or reducing rest periods between exercises. Progression ensures continual challenge and improvement. Listen to your body and progress at a comfortable pace.

## Importance of Rest and Recovery

Stress the significance of rest days in any fitness routine. Muscles need time to recover and grow stronger after workouts. Encourage adequate sleep, hydration, and incorporating restorative activities like yoga or meditation into the routine.

# Celebrating Achievements and Setting Future Goals

Encourage celebrating milestones and progress achieved through consistent workouts. Setting realistic and specific fitness goals, whether it's mastering a new exercise or improving endurance, helps maintain motivation and focus.

## Example Goals:

- Increase wall sit duration by 15 seconds within two weeks.
- Improve balance exercises by reducing reliance on the wall for support.
- Complete a full routine with increased repetitions within a month.

## Conclusion

This final chapter serves as a guide to structuring a personalized wall Pilates routine, understanding the importance of progression, recovery, and maintaining motivation through goal setting.

"Success is the sum of small efforts, repeated day in and day out." - Robert Collier

# Conclusion

## Embrace the Power of Wall Pilates

In the journey toward holistic wellness, the integration of wall Pilates emerges as a transformative ally for women seeking a convenient and effective workout regimen within the comfort of their homes. Through these chapters, we've explored the manifold benefits and versatile exercises that leverage the wall as a supportive tool, sculpting not just the body but also fostering mental resilience and determination.

Wall Pilates, tailored to women's specific fitness needs, nurtures core strength, flexibility, and balance. It forms a holistic approach that transcends physicality, encouraging discipline and perseverance. By laying the foundation with proper form and alignment, we establish a groundwork that ensures safety and maximizes the efficacy of each movement.

The journey through core-strengthening exercises, flexibility enhancement, lower and upper body toning, all while embracing the support of the wall, is a testament to the adaptability and inclusivity of this workout method. Moreover, the flexibility within these routines allows for progression, ensuring a challenge that evolves with individual growth.

Yet, beyond the physical gains, wall Pilates instills a mindset of commitment and celebration. It celebrates each small triumph, whether it's holding a pose a few seconds longer or mastering a challenging movement. It champions the pursuit of personal goals, fostering a sense of accomplishment that extends beyond the confines of the exercise routine.

In the end, wall Pilates transcends mere fitness; it becomes a lifestyle—a choice to prioritize wellness, perseverance, and self-care. Embrace the power of the wall, transform your workout, and relish the journey toward a stronger, more resilient self.

This conclusion encapsulates the holistic benefits of wall Pilates, emphasizing its transformative impact on physical and mental well-being.